The ultimate guide:

How to lose weight

For the first time.

Diana A. Wagaman

Table Of Contents

Chapter one
Chapter Two
Chapter Three
Chapter Four

Chapter one

Why you constantly hungry?

Hunger normally kicks in about two hours from the last time you've eaten a meal.

"You're experiencing bodily indicators of hunger, so your stomach is rumbling, your energy is dropping," On the other hand, emotional hunger doesn't display any bodily indicators. This is when you could experience cravings for particular meals. Zumpano says that around 90% of us indulge in emotional eating. "If you're saying, 'I want chocolate. I want a bag of chips,' that's not hunger," explains Zumpano. "Usually, you're hunting for food and food doesn't satisfy because you're feeding an emotional hunger."

You're not consuming enough protein.
Protein is one of the three macronutrients your body requires (carbohydrates and fats being the other two) to provide you energy. When used

together in a meal, they may help feed your body and keep you feeling full.

For example, a meal high in carbohydrates can cause your sugar to jump and then fall leading to hunger. "When you add protein with a complex carbohydrate, it slows down the pace of glucose. This means you'll have a steady spike and then a gradual decline, which helps you feel more calm and satisfied," And consider beyond meat when seeking for protein to add to your meals. Vegetables and dairy items including yogurt, milk and cheese, eggs, seafood, beans, tofu, seeds, and nuts all include protein.

You're not sleeping well.

If you're not receiving the necessary seven to nine hours of sleep a day, it might contribute to weight gain. Sleep helps control ghrelin, an appetite-stimulating hormone. Not getting enough sleep raises ghrelin, causing you to feel hungry when you're really in need of sleep.

"Sleep is important to help your body system to mend and regenerate," explains Zumpano. "So if you can't obtain sleep during the night, having a little nap or even simply relaxing your body will help."

You're consuming refined carbohydrates.

Watch out for items prepared with refined carbohydrates like white flour or white rice (and yes, things like sweets and baked goods have refined carbs) (and yes, foods like candy and baked goods contain refined carbs).

Those components have been processed and lost many of their minerals and fiber. Eating too many refined carbohydrates doesn't leave you feeling full for long. It boosts your blood sugar and then when it decreases, you're hungry again. "We tend to seek carbohydrates and sweets because every time we consume a little bit, our energy level increases. So when you're weary, you're utilizing your food to produce energy as opposed to your natural sources of energy,"

Your diet is low in fat.

Adding foods that are rich in omega-3 fatty acids like salmon, tuna, sardines, walnuts or flaxseed may assist with your appetite. But if you're missing healthy fat in your diet, it might lead to desiring carbohydrates and meals rich in sugar. So examine that balance of what you eat — it all goes back to wanting those three macronutrients to feel full and content. "Those macronutrients are structured such that we require all three," explains Zumpano. "It's simply modestly boosting your good fats to the point where you experience that sense of satiety."

Your diet needs extra fiber.

Fiber is extremely excellent for so many reasons. But when it comes to hunger, seek meals rich in fiber such as fruits, vegetables, lentils, beans, and oats to help produce appetite-reducing hormones. "Fiber swells in your belly," explains Zumpano. "It enhances that sense of being full earlier."

You're eating while preoccupied.

Popping up a bag of chips while bingeing Netflix may seem like a perfect Friday night for some but try to be more careful of how much food you're eating while following narrative lines. "Mindless eating is when you don't recognize what and how much you're consuming," "You know in your brain that you did eat, but it's almost like rejecting that meal. Your brain doesn't detect that you've eaten."
To prevent mindless eating, portion management is crucial. Zumpano advocates portioning out the necessary number of food before watching TV, driving, or even browsing on your phone.

You're not drinking enough water.

Many of us feel like we're hungry when in reality we're simply thirsty. But before you drink down that fourth cup of coffee, know that that big caramel latte with whipped cream is drying you (not to mention adding unneeded calories) (not to mention adding unnecessary calories).

On the other hand, drinking water throughout the day will keep you hydrated and maybe fend off hunger. "You may be thirsty and not perceive the difference," explains Zumpano. "It's suggested that you consume 64 ounces of water every day."

Chapter Two

You're stressed.

A lot of us will resort to food when we're stressed out – going for that bag of cookies when we're up against a deadline instead of dealing with the root of our feelings. "Find a technique to release the tension without utilizing food to achieve it," recommends Zumpano. "Find something you like and if you feel worried during the day, go away from your desk for five minutes, go outdoors, and get some fresh air."

She also advocates practicing deep breathing or box breathing to naturally relax oneself. Even taking a hot bath, painting your nails, reading or crocheting might help ease tension.

Why you constantly be hungry?

Your body needs energy food, so it's natural to feel hungry if you don't eat for a few hours. But if hunger is something you deal with regularly, some people might benefit from eating every two to three hours and then having a small snack — and by snack, Zumpano means foods like a boiled egg with a cheese stick, whole-grain, low-salt crackers with cheese or an apple with peanut butter.

"Look for whole food selections that offer full carbohydrates, fiber, and protein," she advises.

Why you constantly need food?

If you feel like you're hungry all the time, even after a meal, you're not alone. In a physiological sense, hunger is a signal that your body needs more food. Your stomach may feel empty and grumbly. You can find yourself feeling irritated, or "hangry." You could even feel dizzy or off balance.

But hunger may also be an indication of emotional emptiness. You seek for food in an effort to calm yourself, perhaps out of despair, boredom, even enjoyment. The difficulty is, eating more than your body needs to maintain your regular activities might induce weight growth.

What Is Hunger?

Hunger may be physical, psychological or even a mix of the two. Unfortunately, it may be difficult to discriminate between actual bodily hunger and an emotional urge for food.

Physical hunger: Physical hunger arises when you genuinely need to eat. The stomach is a muscular organ that extends and contracts. When it extends after you take food and fluids, you begin to feel full. A hormone called leptin alerts the body that you're full so you may stop eating.

When your stomach is empty, it contracts or collapses, generating hunger symptoms. Your blood sugar levels plummet, and your stomach generates a hormone called ghrelin, pushing you to eat.

Psychological hunger:

Psychological or emotional hunger is not driven by actual physiological hunger or the demand for nutrients. It arises when you have an emotional attachment to, or longing for, a specific meal owing to habit, stress or environmental stimuli. Unlike actual hunger, emotional hunger creates desires for certain meals – generally something sweet, salty or crunchy.

Chapter Three

Why You're Hungry?

If you often eat a big breakfast only to feel famished an hour later, there might be more behind your growling gut than true hunger. From not getting enough sleep to feeling stressed, here are seven reasons why you could feel.

continuously hungry:

You're not truly hungry. Reaching for the pantry door quickly after eating frequently suggests you're mentally hungry. You're turning to food to deal with undesirable emotions like melancholy, despair and worry. Unfortunately, consuming foods that are salty, sweet or fatty might encourage your brain to produce feel-good chemicals, which simply promotes such eating tendencies. Your best bet: Try the egg test. If you're not hungry for protein like eggs, poultry or beans, you're probably not actually hungry.

Your meals are out of balance. If you're not receiving enough protein, fat and complex carbs, particularly fiber-rich ones, you're likely more likely to feel hungry throughout the day. Each of these nutrients slows digestion and improves feelings of fullness.

On the other hand, consuming too many refined carbs might create blood sugar variations that urge your body to seek more food. You're eating too rapidly. Your body requires around 20 minutes to sense fullness. When you eat slowly and chew your meal completely, your body and brain have time to realize that you're satiated.
Your drugs are the cause.
Medications, such as steroids, anti-seizure medications, some antidepressants and oral contraceptives might cause you to feel hungrier than normal. If you're worried that your drugs are making you feel hungry, speak to your doctor. There may be an option that doesn't generate the same side effects.
You're not getting enough sleep. Sleep and appetite are intricately related. In reality, our

systems manufacture more ghrelin and want more calories when we're not getting enough shut-eye. That's why you frequently feel hungry when you're sleep-deprived. You're truly thirsty. Water not only makes you feel full, it also helps your body absorb the nutrients it obtains from meals. What's more, emotions of thirst might be misinterpreted for hunger. Not sure whether you're hungry or thirsty? Drink a full glass of water before you even contemplate making a meal or snack.

You're stressed. Stress might enhance your appetite. Your body wrongly feels you need more nutrients to satisfy your everyday needs. In reality, the stress hormone cortisol may throw your blood sugar levels into a spiral, leading to hunger and food cravings.
Satisfy Your Hunger

Whether your hunger is physical, psychological, or any mix of the two, it's crucial to get to the core of insatiable hunger - and limit overeating. A few essential strategies:

Wait it out. Distract yourself from your desires with a non-eating activity like a guided meditation, a walk outside or a phone call with a friend. If you can wait even three minutes, there's a strong chance the urge will pass.

Strive for equilibrium. Sometimes hunger between meals suggests your diet is low in protein, fat and fiber, which require longer to digest. You'll feel full for longer after eating a spinach salad topped with garbanzo beans, hard-boiled eggs, and nuts or seeds than you would after noshing on a plate of spaghetti.

Keep a dietary journal. Awareness is the first step toward transformation. You can get there by tracking your dietary consumption. In the log, record the kind and quantity of food you consume, the date and the time. You may also handle queries like: Am I hungry? Why am I eating? Where am I eating? Am I doing anything else while eating? What is my mood? After many days, you may be able to notice specific trends in your food consumption and make modifications appropriately.

If you feel hungry all the time and are consuming more calories than you need, take a step back and analyze what's causing your appetite.

Are you thirsty? Overtired? Stressed? Do you need extra fiber in your diet? Whatever the cause, reach first for whole fruits and veggies, or a hard-boiled egg, before you attempt to quell those urges with processed meals and snacks. Still can't get to the bottom of your constant hunger? Talk to a health professional. Constant hunger might be an indicator of health disorders like diabetes, hyperthyroidism, depression and pregnancy. It's crucial to rule out medical issues while treating those hunger pains.

How Do I Know When I Am Hungry or Full?

To know when you are hungry and when you are full. During your meal or snack (at about halfway is best), take time out to check in with your body. Does the food still taste good? Do you want more? Are you still hungry? If not, then stop eating. Before, during, and after a meal use this scale to help you know your hunger and fullness cues.

At 0, you are starving. You've gone too long without eating (6-8 hours) and are probably irritated and unpleasant. You could be feeling queasy or dizzy, or you may have a headache.

At 1, you are hungry. All you can think about is how hungry you are. You can only think about what you want to eat. When you do eat it is probable that you will overeat.

At 2, you are too hungry. You are probably irritated. You may have a headache. Your stomach could be hurting by now. It has probably been 4 or more hours since you last ate.

At 3, you are feeling hunger pains. It's time to eat. Your body is sending you the natural indications that it needs nourishment. This is a decent number to start eating–wait much longer and you will be too hungry. It has probably been roughly 2-3 hours since you last ate.

At 4, your appetite is only beginning to stir. There is a sensation of emptiness in your gut. This might be an ideal time to eat. You may have eaten roughly 2 hours ago.

At 5, you are neutral. You aren't hungry or full-this feeling occurs between mealtimes. If you experience this and want to eat, it is not due to hunger-you may want to eat out of boredom or tension.

At 6, you are simply pleased. You aren't hungry anymore, but presumably will be in approximately 2 hours. There is more space for food, yet you still feel light and invigorated. This is a nice spot to complete a meal or snack.

At 7, you are 'just right. You have eaten your fill of the meal you desired. You are no longer hungry and you probably won't need to eat again for around 3 hours. This is also a nice spot to complete a meal or snack.

At 8, you had a couple of bites too much. You ate a couple more bites since it was there or tasted delicious. You can feel a touch bloated like you need to remove the top button of your jeans. You may not be hungry for another 4-5 hours.

At 9, you are stuffed. You have gone overboard. Your dinner has gone beyond the point of enjoyment and you now feel uncomfortable. You may feel a little numb or tired. You will not be hungry for approximately 6 hours.

At 10, you feel nauseous. You feel uncomfortable to the point of pain. You may need to lie down until you feel better. You should anticipate feeling hungry again in about 7-8 hours.

Chapter Four

Weight loss challenge.

How to reduce weight safely, It's crucial to remember that the purpose of an exercise challenge is to feel better. You should push yourself, but not at the price of your whole physical, emotional, and psychological well-being. If you are new to working out, consult with a healthcare practitioner before beginning a new program. Going too long between eating and overeating at mealtimes makes it harder

Weight reduction should occur from healthy food and increased activity practices. Avoid developing a deprivation attitude, where you do not allow yourself to consume particular foods even if you desire them.

Eating a range of healthful meals is far healthier for your body than restricting yourself. Choose nutrient-dense meals like fruits and vegetables when you can and minimize overly processed items.

You must allow your body time to relax and recuperate between exercises. Take at least 1 day every week to rest, with no rigorous activity. Without any rest, you risk injury and you may not be able to work out as well since your muscles may be weary. This might cause your results to halt, or plateau.

You may lessen the likelihood of this happening by including rest days into your schedule and obtaining great sleep so that your body can replenish itself. It is also crucial that you are receiving adequate protein. It can your body to heal, develop, and keep lean mass.

The Academy of Nutrition and Dietetics, Dietitians of Canada, and the American College of Sports Medicine recommend 1.2 to 2.0 grams of protein per kg body weight per day for athletes depending on training. In contrast, the Dietary Reference Intake Report Trusted Sourcerecommends that sedentary adults consume 0.8 grams of protein per kg body weight or 0.36 grams per pound.

While those guidelines are helpful, it is vital to also focus on eating protein throughout the day. You should also keep your macronutrient intake balanced by consuming a healthy ratio of carbohydrates, fat, and protein at each meal. This can also help to manage your weight.

Workplace weight loss challenge ideas
With these fitness and nutritional suggestions in mind, there are various ways to get straight into a challenge with your co-workers. Use these ideas as inspiration to build a challenge that drives your group.

1. Mileage.
One method to establish a workplace challenge with your co-workers is to designate a particular distance for walking or jogging. Choose a realistic amount of time and challenge yourself to conquer a certain amount of miles during that period. For example, each member may be assigned with walking or running a particular number of kilometers every week. Keep in mind

your fitness level and that of your co-workers. The person who remains consistent or improves their fitness level wins

2. Body scan.

In a body scan challenge, each individual has their body composition documented before and after the competition. A typical body scan includes: a body fat percentage test\body mass index (BMI) calculation\height and weight measurement\measurement of the places on your body where you hold the most mass (abdomen, hips, thigh, etc) (abdomen, hips, thigh, etc.)
At the end of a given time, check the results to see if you have achieved your goal. Then celebrate as a group with something fun, like taking a virtual cooking class together.

3. Workout logs

Keeping a workout log is an easy way to encourage a group of co-workers to become more active. It's a wonderful approach to keep track of which body parts you have worked on over the week so particular regions aren't overworked. It is a wonderful method to remember yourself to integrate rest days into your program. Additionally, it might enable you to monitor your development as you become stronger. It may be an incredibly useful tool, particularly for beginners.

4. Head-to-head contests

One method to spark a group's competitive spirit is to arrange a competition. One approach is to do several exercises over many weeks, where participants are teamed up against one another. In situations of walking and running workouts, it may be the individual who completes the activity in a quicker time that goes on to the next round. The last head-to-head exercise selects the champion.

5. Benchmark workouts

Benchmarks are sets for the same exercises done weeks or months apart. They are meant to monitor development and help you gauge your advancement.

For example, your group conducts a specific exercise on January 1, then logs how each member finishes. Each participant continues to practice for the remainder of the month. Then on February 1, your group conducts the same program and compares those outcomes to the January 1 session.

To choose a winner in this situation, the scores are compared and reviewed to find out who made the greatest improvement in a month.

The bottom line.
When putting up a weight reduction challenge, it's crucial not to ignore self-esteem. In a setting where emotions might build, your group should keep focused on achieving progress (even in little stages), not necessarily on winning. The main thing to remember is that you want to make your exercises interesting and build a habit. Ultimately, you want to feel your best without being attached to the number on a scale